BLOOD PRESSURE MANAGEMENT:

Hypertension and Hypotension

A Guide for Patients, Nurses and other Healthcare Professionals

Solomon Barroa, R.N.

Copyright 2012

All rights reserved. No part of this book may be reproduced by any means, electronic, mechanical, photocopying, recording, scanning or otherwise without permission from the author. The author reserves the right not to be responsible for the correctness, completeness or quality of the information provided. Liability claims regarding damage caused by the use of any information provided, including any kind of information that is incomplete or incorrect, will be rejected. The information contained in this book does not constitute medical advice, and is for information and educational purposes only. Consult your health care provider regarding health concerns.

To Dr. Lee Robbins, Mary Ann, Rosario, Vicente, Benedicto, and Robert.

PURPOSE:

The intention of this book is to educate the layperson and healthcare professionals about blood pressure iregularities and support them in moving towards a more effective role in managing the situation. This includes the many important interactions with medical professionals as well as other providers in the vast industry of diagnosis, services, supplements and information for blood pressure irregularities.

In order to do so, this book provides substantial technical information about the body, its normal functions and how they are affected by blood pressure, the mechanism and symptomatology of blood pressure deregulation and considerable practical advice regarding treatment and management. Some individuals reading the book will want to pursue all of these areas with equal intensity; others may find their needs focus more heavily on the nature of the disease itself or how to manage it. The Introduction and Table of Contents will assist readers in choosing whether to read the material from cover to cover or to focus upon particular issues covered in the various chapters. The Searchable nature of e-books will also assist readers to look up a particular topic of interest or importance to them. The reader should feel free to choose the sections of the text of greatest relevance and usefulness to you.

It is my intent as an author to be helpful to all readers and to encourage them to use this wide-ranging material in the manner that most strongly meets their needs. However, this book is not intended to constitute medical advice. The reader has the responsibility to consult a healthcare provider or another healthcare professional. The author welcomes your comments and suggestions and can be reached at

solomon_barroa@yahoo.com

or at http://www.amazon.com/Solomon-Barroa-RN/e/B00AV3V34S /

PLEASE DON'T USE THIS TEXT FOR MEDICAL ADVICE OR DIAGNOSIS.

READING BEYOND THIS NOTICE IMPLIES YOU'VE READ AND AGREE TO THE ABOVE DISCLAIMER FOR YOUR OWN SAFETY. THANK YOU.

Introduction

The meaning of life is mysterious. Each of us has our own way of life. It is either a busy and stressed lifestyle or a carefree one. As we live, we notice changes in our bodies arising primarily because of stress and aging. These changes sometimes result in deterioration from our previous level of functionality. Bodily diseases are another major culprit for deterioration. The process of aging is not avoidable and diseases are a common occurrence. These diseases are either acute or chronic. One of these diseases is a defect in blood pressure regulation; the presence of either low or high blood pressure result in risks to our health.

This book will enable the reader to understand and manage fluctuations in blood pressure. It has chapters designed to give the important information that will make readers ready to take charge of their own condition. Medical terminologies are explained in the Glossary section of this book.

Chapter 1 is about defining and understanding the basic concepts of blood pressure. The heart, blood vessels and different factors affecting the blood circulation maintain the blood pressure. Blood pressure is a result of the heart's activity. This chapter discusses the different structures of the body that play a role in blood pressure.

Chapter 2 talks about the regulation of the blood pressure. The regulators of blood pressure are the cardiovascular center of the brain, the hormones of the body, neural receptors and bodily tissues. These structures of the body are interconnected to each other and function interdependently. This chapter provides the reader with an understanding of the physiological processes that are involved in the regulation of the blood pressure.

Chapter 3 is about the physical aspects of the body that affect blood pressure. These factors are peripheral resistance and elasticity of the blood vessels, blood volume and cardiac output. The blood is pumped by the heart, passed along the blood vessels and oxygenated in the capillaries. Any defect in the process will affect blood pressure regulation. This chapter elaborates the effects of these factors on the blood pressure.

Chapter 4 talks about the drugs and medications for blood pressure. Drugs and medication are classified into antihypertensive and antihypotensive. The antihypertensive drugs are used to lessen overly high blood pressure and antihypotensive drugs are used to increase overly low blood pressure. This chapter will provides the reader information regarding the different drug classifications, their generic names, the adverse effects and contraindications.

Chapter 5 is about the facts regarding hypertension. The state of excessively high blood pressure is asymptomatic for the majority of people. Ordinarily only in the third stage more severe stage do symptoms show up causing organ failure. This chapter contains information regarding the classification, diagnosis, causes, stages and complications of hypertension.

Chapter 6 talks about the facts regarding hypotension. A blood pressure below the normally acceptable range is called hypotension. It is usually associated with symptoms. This chapter will provide the reader the information regarding the causes and symptoms of hypotension. It also discusses essential facts about orthostatic hypotension.

Chapter 7 is about measuring your own blood pressure. Being in charge and taking an active role in self-care is a good practice in managing blood pressure irregularities. The ability to monitor one's own blood pressure saves time and effort for the individual who undertakes self-monitoring. This chapter will provide the reader with the steps for using the different types of blood pressure monitors and some rationale for the specific steps in each procedure.

Chapter 8 is the last chapter of this book. It talks about blood pressure management. After the diagnosis of either hypotension or a hypertension, a diagnosed person should participate and play an active role in doing self-care. This chapter provides the reader with salient points about blood pressure management such as lifestyle modification, medications, physical activity, dietary intake, stress management, smoking cessation, weight reduction, alcohol reduction and health information.

Table of Contents

Chapter 1 The Heart and Blood Pressure..................9

The Heart..................9
Blood Circulation..................10
Blood Vessels..................10
Blood Pressure..................11

Chapter 2 Regulation of Blood Pressure..................12

The Brain Regulates Blood Pressure..................12
The Neural Receptors Regulates Blood Pressure..................12
The Hormones Regulate Blood Pressure..................13
The Body Autoregulates Blood Pressure..................13

Chapter 3 The Physical Factors in the Body that Affects Blood Pressure 14

The Peripheral Resistance of the Blood Vessels..................14
The Elasticity of the Blood Vessel..................14
The Volume of Blood..................15
The Cardiac Output of the Heart..................15

Chapter 4 Drugs and Medications for Blood Pressure..................16

Antihypertensive Medications..................16
Antihypotensive Medication..................18

Chapter 5 High Blood Pressure: Facts About Hypertension..................20

Classification of Hypertension..................20
Diagnosing Hypertension..................21
Causes of High Blood Pressure..................21
Hypertensive Crisis..................24
Complications of Uncontrolled Hypertension..................24

Chapter 6 Low Blood Pressure: Facts About Hypotension..................26

Causes of Low Blood Pressure..................26
Symptoms of Hypotension..................27

Chapter 7 Measuring Your Own Blood Pressure..................28

Monitoring Blood Pressure Using Either A Mercury Or An Aneroid Blood Pressure Monitor *28*
The Procedure for Taking Blood Pressure using a Mercury and Aneroid Blood Pressure Monitor *28*
The Procedure for Taking Blood Pressure using an Electronic Blood Pressure Monitor *29*

Chapter 8 Blood Pressure Management 31

Managing Dietary Intake *31*
Managing A Physically Active Body *31*
Managing Smoking Cessation *32*
Managing Stress and Pressure in Daily Life *32*
Managing Blood Pressure through Medications *33*
Managing Weight Loss *33*
Managing Alcohol Consumption *34*
Managing Health Information *34*
Managing Lifestyle Modification *35*

Glossary 36

References 40

Index 41

Chapter 1 The Heart and Blood Pressure

Knowledge about the cardiovascular system and its structure is the initial step in understanding blood pressure. The cardiovascular system is composed of different structures that regulate blood flow throughout the body. This chapter discusses the heart, blood vessels and the two types of blood circulation. We will name and describe these structures and help you to understand the role they play in blood pressure regulation – and the effects produced on the system by hypertension and hypotension.

The Heart

The heart is an organ located at the back of the sternum and in front of the vertebral column. It is likened in size to a fist. At least two thirds of the total lies in the left portion of the thoracic cavity. It is very muscular in nature and distributes blood to the entire body.

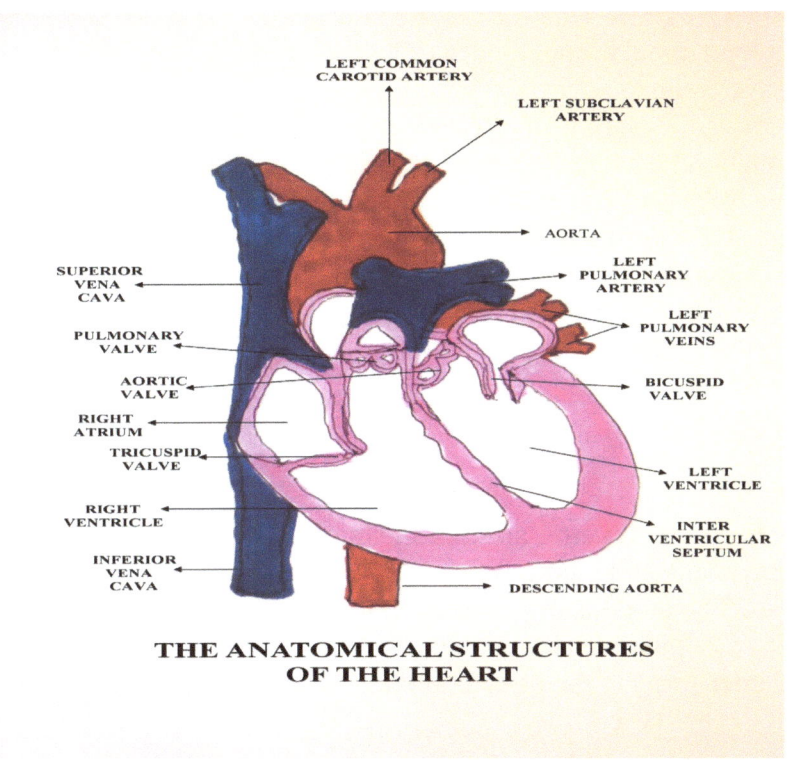

THE ANATOMICAL STRUCTURES OF THE HEART

The heart is composed of four chambers and four valves. The four chambers are called the two upper atriums and the two lower ventricles. Atriums and ventricles are divided into left and right sub-chambers. The right atrium receives deoxygenated blood from the body through major veins that are connected to the heart. These veins are called superior and inferior vena cava.

The right ventricle receives the deoxygenated blood from the right atrium and passes it to the lungs for oxygenation through the pulmonary arteries. Both left and right lungs process the oxygenation of blood through the exchange of oxygen and carbon dioxide gases. The left atrium receives oxygenated blood from the lungs through the pulmonary veins. This oxygenated blood is passed to the left ventricle for distribution throughout the body.

The aorta is the major artery, which distributes the oxygenated blood. It branches into smaller arteries. The four valves of the heart are atrioventricular valves and semilunar valves. The atrioventricular valves are called tricuspid and bicuspid. These valves are located between the atriums and ventricles. The pressure of the blood in the chambers causes the valves to open and permits it to flow. The semilunar valves are called aortic and pulmonic. These valves prevent the backflow of blood into the heart and permit the flow into the arteries. The cardiac output is the amount of blood that is pumped by the heart. Heart rate is the rate of contraction by the heart.

Blood Circulation

The process of blood circulation includes two processes. These processes are called pulmonary and systemic.

Pulmonary circulation takes place between the heart and the lungs. The deoxygenated blood is received by the right side of the heart and passed to the lungs for oxygenation. Oxygen is added and carbon dioxide is removed through the process of blood oxygenation in the lungs. This systemic circulation of the blood is processed by both lungs and the left side of the heart. Through this process, oxygenated blood is distributed to the different parts of the body.

Blood Vessels

The blood vessels comprise veins, arteries and capillaries. The veins of the circulatory system carry deoxygenated blood from the different parts of the body. They transport blood to the heart. The blood is oxygenated in the lungs after passing through the right side of the heart. The pulmonary vein is the only vein that carries oxygenated blood from the lungs. The larger veins in the body branch to smaller ones called venules. These venules connect to capillaries.

The capillaries, microscopic in size, function for exchanging body nutrients and wastes. This is also where the blood is oxygenated. The blood travels to the arterioles after it has been oxygenated. The arterioles are small branches of arteries that connect to the big arteries. The constriction and dilation of the blood vessels is known to directly affect blood pressure.

Blood Pressure

The pressure that is put forth by the circulating blood upon the walls of the blood vessel is called the blood pressure. It is also known as the arterial pressure. It is subdivided into two specific types. These are **systolic** and **diastolic** pressures. The systolic pressure is the highest pressure in the arteries. It occurs when the heart contracts and the blood is being ejected into the aorta and the arteries. It is **the upper number** in a blood pressure measurement. The diastolic pressure is the lowest pressure occurring when the heart is relaxed. The blood returns to the heart from the vena cava and the veins. It is **the lower number** in a blood pressure measurement. The elevation and lowering of the blood pressure is caused by numerous factors as discussed in the chapters on hypertension and hypotension.

Chapter 2 Regulation of Blood Pressure

The blood pressure is regulated by the brain, hormones, neural receptors and autoregulatory processes. Effective blood pressure regulation enables the individual to live either asymptomatically or with mild symptoms. However the blood pressure can become either excessively elevated or overly lowered. If there is extensive deregulation above or below the desirable range of blood pressure, symptoms become profound. The nature, presence and degree of symptoms differ from one person to another.

The Brain Regulates Blood Pressure

The brain regulates blood pressure through its cardiovascular center. It is located in the medulla oblongata. The cardiovascular center of the brain regulates heart rate, the contraction of the heart, the dilation and constriction of blood vessels. This part of the brain receives input from sensory receptors, the cerebral cortex, the limbic system and the hypothalamus.

The sensory receptors are proprioceptors, baroreceptors and chemoreceptors. The proprioceptors are sensory receptors that monitor the movement of the muscles and joints of the body. Baroreceptors monitor the changes in the walls of the blood vessels. The chemoreceptors monitor the concentration of different chemicals in the blood such as carbon dioxide. The cardiovascular center of the brain processes these inputs into outputs.

The autonomic nervous system receives the outputs. It is comprised of the sympathetic and parasympathetic divisions. The sympathetic components of the autonomic nervous system will stimulate the heart rate and increase the contraction of the heart while the parasympathetic components will do the opposite. Furthermore, the sympathetic components will stimulate the muscles of the vein causing constriction that leads to increased blood pressure. The cardiovascular center of the brain also controls the vasomotor tone of the smooth muscles of the arterioles causing contraction and constriction.

The Neural Receptors Regulates Blood Pressure

The two most common neural receptors are baroreceptor and chemoreceptor. They produce a reflex reaction that sends impulses to the cardiovascular center of the brain. The baroreceptors are located in the arch of the aorta and in the carotid sinuses. In the event of an elevated blood pressure, these baroreceptors are stretched. The cardiovascular center reacts by increasing parasympathetic stimulation resulting to a decreased cardiac output. This process normalizes the blood pressure. The chemoreceptors are located in the carotid sinuses and arch of the aorta. They detect chemical changes in blood such as that of increases in either carbon dioxide or hydrogen ions. Impulses will be sent to cardiovascular center of the brain regarding these changes. The result would be constriction of the muscles of the blood vessels that ultimately increase the blood pressure.

The Hormones Regulate Blood Pressure

The major hormones that regulate blood pressure are antidiuretic hormones, epinephrine and norepinephrine, atrial natriuretic peptide and the renin-angiotensin-aldosterone hormonal system (RAAS). The antidiuretic hormones are produced in the hypothalamus of the brain. These hormones are also called vasopressin. They are released from the posterior part of the pituitary gland. These hormones produce vasoconstriction resulting in an increased blood pressure. Epinephrine and norepinephrine are released from the adrenal medulla of the adrenal gland as a response to sympathetic stimulation. They increase cardiac output and constriction of blood vessels that leads to an elevated blood pressure.

The renin-angiotensin-aldosterone hormonal system (RAAS) is a complex process involved in regulating blood pressure. Whenever there is a decrease in the volume of blood that is supplied to the kidneys, renin is secreted. The enzyme renin catalyzes the angiotensinogen peptide and converts it to angiotensin 1. The angiotensin converting enzyme catalyzes angiotensin 1 and converts it to angiotensin 2. The aldosterone hormone will be released by angiotensin 2 resulting to vasoconstriction of the arterioles. It also increases the reabsorption of sodium by the kidney. This reabsorption takes place in the distal tubules of the kidney. Water is also reabsorbed as a consequence of sodium reabsorption. The process increases the blood volume and blood pressure. The atrial natriuretic peptide hormone is released from the atria of the heart. It causes vasodilation of the arterioles and the excretion of sodium and water in the kidneys. The effect is a decrease in blood pressure.

The Body Autoregulates Blood Pressure

The autoregulation of blood pressure is done by the body tissues. The blood flow is automatically adjusted to match the body's metabolic demands. The blood vessels are either constricted or dilated. Whenever there is a physical change in the temperature of the environment, autoregulation takes place. Warm temperature causes vasodilation of the blood vessels and the opposite happens with cold temperature. There are also chemical elements that are released by blood cells and body tissues leading to a vasodilatory effect. These chemicals are potassium, hydrogen, adenosine phosphate and nitric oxide. When the autoregulation is functioning well, the blood pressure is kept within a range described as "normal blood pressure".

Chapter 3 The Physical Factors in the Body that Affects Blood Pressure

The first chapter of this book discussed the different structures of the body that play a role in the level and variation of blood pressure. The physical make up of the body structures, the blood volume and cardiac output are major factors that cause the changes in the blood pressure.

The Peripheral Resistance of the Blood Vessels

The blood vessel is the structure through which the blood passes. Resistance occurs within the vessel due to the friction between the blood and the walls of the blood vessels and resistance increases the degree of blood pressure needed to move the blood through these vessels.

There are at least four known factors that lead to the peripheral resistance within these vessels. The first factor is the diameter of the blood vessel. The diameter of the vessels must accommodate the volume of blood passing through. The diameter of the vessels decreases in the peripheral blood vessels, which produces an increase in the resistance to the blood flow leading to an elevation in pressure. The second factor is the vasomotor fibers in the blood vessels. It is composed of sympathetic nerve fibers that activate the muscle of the blood vessel. It releases a neurotransmitter such as norepinephrine that constricts the muscle of the vessel causing resistance and elevated pressure.

The third factor is the viscosity, thickness, of the blood. The circulating blood can become viscous because of the hematocrit or red blood cells. Viscous blood will have less plasma fluid and more of the red blood cells or hematocrit. This leads to increase resistance and elevated pressure. The fourth factor is the total length of the blood vessel. The presence of more adipose tissue tends to lengthen the size of the blood vessels, which increases the resistance in the peripheries.

The Elasticity of the Blood Vessel

The smooth muscle in the wall of an artery is elastic and recoils to accommodate the blood that is passing through. It stretches and propels the blood even when the ventricles are relaxed. When the artery loses the ability to stretch and expand, it produces a large amount of pressure while the artery itself becomes weaker and weaker. This results in an extremely elevated blood pressure. Atherosclerosis is an example of such a condition in which the arterial wall thickens due to the accumulation of low density lipoproteins such as cholesterol and triglycerides.

The Volume of Blood

The volume of blood passing through the blood vessel is directly related to the degree of resistance it creates. A lower volume of blood passing through the vessel correlates with less resistance. Hypovolemia is a condition in which there is significantly low volume of blood. It occurs when there is hemorrhage and extensive burns. In stage three of such hypovolemic shock the blood drops significantly. Less blood is circulated than needed to maintain tissue perfusion. It is a medical emergency. The objective of medical intervention is to increase the blood pressure and stabilize it within normal levels.

The Cardiac Output of the Heart

The heart pumps blood to the arteries. It is known as the cardiac output. Low blood pressure results from a low cardiac output. A defect in the muscles or in the valves of the heart will produce a deficient cardiac output.

Negative inotropic medication weakens the ability of the heart muscles to contract. Drugs such as calcium channel blockers are negative inotropic agents. In circumstances in which cardiac output decrease to an excessive degree such drugs need to be withdrawn and positive inotropic agents such as digoxin may be given to maintain the contractility of the heart muscles.

Chapter 4 Drugs and Medications for Blood Pressure

Hypertension is a condition of elevated blood pressure above the level considered acceptable by the medical profession, while the state of hypotension is a low blood pressure that is below the acceptable level. There are two common classifications of drugs and medications that prescribed to manage blood pressure. These drugs are either antihypertensive or antihypotensive.

Antihypertensive Medications

Diuretics are drugs that promote the process of diuresis [an increase in water retention] resulting in an increase in urination. The classifications of diuretics are thiazides, potassium sparing, carbonic anhydrase inhibitors, xanthines and loop diuretics.

Commonly prescribed thiazide diuretics are bendroflumethiazide and hydrochlorothiazide. These drugs inhibit the reabsorption of sodium at the distal convoluted tubules of the kidneys. The common adverse effects are muscle cramps and weakness, thirst, hypotension, confusion, fatigue, hypokalemia (low levels of potassium) and gastrointestinal disturbances such as nausea and vomiting. The potassium sparing diuretics that are commonly prescribed are spironolactone, triamterene and amiloride. These drugs function to inhibit the exchange between sodium and potassium in the collecting ducts of the kidneys. The adverse effects are hyperkalemia (elevated levels of potassium) resulting in arrhythmia and muscle weakness, and metabolic acidosis that results in seizures, coma, lethargy and breathing difficulties.

The carbonic anhydrase inhibitors diuretics that are commonly prescribed are azetazolamide and dorzolamide. These drugs function to inhibit the secretion of hydrogen ions in the proximal tubules of the kidneys. The common adverse effects are hypokalemia and central nervous system disturbances such as seizures and coma. The commonly prescribed xanthine diuretics are theophylline, theobromine and caffeine. These drugs function to inhibit reabsorption of sodium and increase the glomerular filtration rate of the kidneys. Theophylline is not generally recommended because of the toxic effects to the cardiovascular system.

Over all, the general adverse effects of diuretics are imbalances in the potassium levels in the blood, hypercalcemia (elevated levels of calcium), hyponatremia (lower levels of sodium), hyperuricemia (excessive uric acid in the blood) and orthostatic hypotension (postural hypotension). Diuretics are contraindicated for people with gout because it will elevate the uric acid in the blood.

A health teaching regarding the adverse effects of diuretics should be done by the healthcare provider. Monitoring other bodily reactions such as weight changes and neurological deficits is needed due to concern over potential negative effects of the drug to the body. Constant updates to the healthcare providers regarding bodily changes are important so that necessary adjustment in the dosage can be promptly done.

Beta blockers are drugs that block the beta receptors of the sympathetic nervous system such as epinephrine and other stress hormones. Aside from hypertension, these drugs are used for many other diseases such as congestive heart failure and cardiac arrhythmia. The commonly prescribed beta blockers are atenolol, metoprolol and carvedilol. The adverse effects are bradycardia (decrease in heart rate), bronchospasm (narrowing of the bronchioles), insomnia (inability to sleep), fatigue, gastrointestinal (stomach and intestines) disturbances such as nausea and vomiting, dizziness and among others. Beta blockers are contraindicated for asthma and depression. Always consult the healthcare provider regarding the adverse effects of these drugs.

ACE inhibitors are drugs that inhibit the angiotensin converting enzyme. These drugs block the conversion of angiotensin 1 to angiotensin 2. It results in the vasodilation of the blood vessel thereby lowering blood pressure. The commonly prescribed ACE inhibitors are captopril, enalapril, lisinopril and benazipril. The adverse effects are dry cough, angioedema, hyperkalemia and kidney impairment and among others. Hyperkalemia is due to the low aldosterone levels that is suppose to excrete potassium. The aldosterone levels are decreased by the suppression of angiotensin 2. Dry cough and angioedema are results of the increases in the bradykinin levels in the body. Bradykinin is a receptor that produces vasodilation and eventually lowers the blood pressure. ACE inhibitor is contraindicated during pregnancy and with kidney diseases.

Alpha blockers are drugs that blocked the alpha adrenergic receptors of the nervous sytem. These drugs are also used for treating anxiety and panic disorders. The most commonly prescribed alpha blockers are terazosin and doxazosin. Some of the adverse effects are dry mouth, fatigue and postural hypotension. A special precaution is given to older people because of the decrease capability of the body to metabolize the drug.

Calcium channel blockers are drugs that block the movement of calcium in the different transport mechanisms of the body such as in intracellular networks. These drugs function to reduce the muscular contraction of the heart and the smooth muscles of the blood vessels. They eventually results in a decreased contractility of the heart and the vasodilation of the blood vessels leading to a lower blood pressure. There are two classes of calcium channel blockers, the dihydropyridines and the non-dihydropyridines. The commonly prescribed drugs under the dihydropyridines classification are amlodipine and nicardipine, while diltiazem and verapamil are commonly prescribed drugs under the non-dihydropyridines classification. Some of the adverse effects are edema of the legs and ankle, tachycardia and headache.

Vasodilators are drugs that promote the relaxation of the smooth muscles of the blood vessels. They result in a decrease in the peripheral resistance causing a lower blood pressure. The commonly prescribed vasodilators are hydralazine and minoxidil. The adverse effects are tachycardia, headache and among others. These drugs are contraindicated for autoimmune disorders such as systemic lupus erythematosus.

Renin inhibitors are drugs that inhibit the conversion of angiotensinogen to angiotensin 1. Aliskiren is the most widely prescribed renin inhibitor. The adverse effects are cough, edema of the dermis and subcutaneous tissues, and gastrointestinal disturbances such as diarrhea.

Central alpha agonists are drugs that stimulate the alpha receptors in the brain. The alpha receptors will expand the blood vessels and eventually lower the peripheral resistance. The commonly prescribed central alpha agonists are methyldopa and clonidine. The adverse effects are dry mouth, fatigue, postural hypotension and among others. These drugs are contraindicated for people with hepatitis and cirrhosis.

Angiotensin receptor blockers are drugs that block the activation of the angiotensin 2 receptors. The result is vasodilation. The most commonly prescribed angiotensin receptor blockers are losartan and valsartan. The adverse effects are hyperkalemia, dizziness and among others. These drugs are contraindicated during pregnancy.

The antihypertensive drugs are prescribed with a combination of two drugs or more in lower doses. The combination could be a diuretic and a blocker or two blockers at the same time. It is crucial to monitor older adults while taking these drugs because of the adverse effects such as orthostatic hypotension that leads to fall incidents. The occurrence of adverse effect will differ from one person to another. Some people will be asymptomatic while other people will have more than the usual adverse effects. It is prudent to research and ask questions regarding these drugs and medications from the healthcare provider before taking it.

Antihypotensive Medication

Vasopressors are drugs that constrict the blood vessels. The effect of these drugs is the elevation of the blood pressure due to the increase resistance in the flow of blood along the blood vessels. The commonly classified vasopressors are sympathomimetics. Sympathomimetics are drugs that imitate the effects of catecholamines in the sympathetic nervous system.

Catecholamines are neurotransmitters of the nervous system. The most abundant catecholamines are epinephrine, dopamine and norepinephrine. The commonly prescribed symphatomimetics are dobutamine, dopamine, epinephrine, noradrenaline hydrotartrate, phenylephrine, and ephedrine hydrochloride. The adverse effects are palpitation, tachycardia, headache, hypertension and among others. These drugs are contraindicated for people with coronary artery disease because it may precipitate myocardial ischemia (decreased oxygen of the heart muscles), cerebrovascular accident (stroke) and myocardial infarction (heart attack).

The occurrence of adverse effect for taking antihypotensive differs from one person to another. Some people will be asymptomatic while other people will have more than the usual adverse effects. It is prudent to research and ask questions regarding these drugs before committing to their continued use.

Chapter 5 High Blood Pressure: Facts About Hypertension

Hypertension is a chronic condition in which the blood pressure in the arteries is constantly above the normally acceptable range. It is also known as the silent killer because of the absence of symptoms in the majority of people who have hypertension. The previous chapters informed us that elevated blood pressure is due to peripheral resistance, vasoconstriction, cardiac diseases and among other reasons.

Classification of Hypertension

Hypertension can be classified as primary and secondary. Primary hypertension is a kind of hypertension that arises from everyday life as the body undergoes the process of adaptation to the environment and aging. Factors such as the certain physical environments, dietary intake and sedentary lifestyle contribute to its development. Primary hypertension is also known as essential hypertension. Secondary hypertension, by contrast, is a result of a bodily disorder and may arise due to certain drugs and medications.

Primary hypertension has four stages. The stages are categorized according to the blood pressure reading obtained from a person. The intention of defining different stages is to provide medical personnel with guidelines for whether, when and how vigorously to attempt corrective intervention such as medication or lifestyle changes as discussed in other sections of this book.

A reading of 120 – 139 mmhg (millimiters of mercury) for systolic and 80-89 mmhg for diastolic means that the person is in the prehypertension stage, a reading of 140 – 159 mmhg for systolic and 90-99 mmhg for diastolic means stage 1 of hypertension, a reading of 160 mmhg for systolic and 100 mmhg for diastolic means stage 2 of hypertension and a reading of 180 mmhg for systolic and 110 mmhg for diastolic means that the individual is in hypertensive crisis.

Secondary hypertension as noted above is a result of a bodily disorder or from certain drugs and medications. Examples of body disorders and conditions which can give rise to secondary hypertension include kidney diseases, tumors of the adrenal glands, Cushing's syndrome (hypercortisolism), imbalances in the thyroid glands secretion, obesity and coarctation of the aorta (narrowing of the aorta). Drugs such as MAOI (monoamine oxidase inhibitor), TCA (tricyclic antidepressant), amphetamines, ephedra, corticosteroids, epoetin, PPA (phenylpropanolamine) and herbal remedies also can elevate blood pressure sometimes to a damaging level.

Diagnosing Hypertension

To confirm a diagnosis of hypertension, a consistent elevated blood pressure reading equal to or greater than 140 mmhg for the systolic and 90 mmhg or higher for the diastolic must have occurred in three separate measurements at one monthly intervals. Once a person is confirmed to have hypertension, the next step would be to classify the type of hypertension. If the person is classified to have a secondary hypertension, laboratory tests, medical history, physical examination and medical procedures are done to check for further evidence of causal factors. Laboratory tests include urinalysis, kidney function tests and echocardiogram. Medical procedures such as electrocardiogram and chest x-ray are also ordered. Furthermore, an assessment of all the prescribed drugs is undertaken.

The process of measuring hypertension requires using a mercury sphygmomanometer. There had been technological advances recently leading to aneroid and electronic blood pressure monitors. These newer blood pressure monitors were designed to prevent mercurial pollution in the environment and for convenient use and applicability in the patient's own home. The accuracy of results from these newer devices is still being debated.

ABPM (ambulatory blood pressure monitoring) is also performed to confirm the diagnosis of hypertension. It is useful for people who have drug resistant hypertension, white coat hypertension, episodic hypertension and borderline hypertension. White coat hypertension is blood pressure elevated in a physician's office because of anxiety. The process of ABPM is performed with the patient wearing an inflatable cuff around the arm with the monitor placed in a holster around the waistline for 24 or 48 hours during their normal life activities. The cuff automatically inflates at predetermined times. Through the ABPM, blood pressure is measured every 15 to 30 minutes during the day and 30 to 60 minutes during the night.

Causes of High Blood Pressure

The causes and reasons for hypertension are complex and broad. It is a combination of multiple factors. Symptoms usually do not appear until the late stages. The causes can be any or most of the following: metabolic syndrome, genetics, aging, sedentary lifestyle, obesity, diseases, excessive alcohol intake, smoking, stress, certain medications and dietary intake.

Metabolic Syndrome is the existence of a number of factors that directly relate to a metabolism disorder such as hypertriglyceridemia (higher than normal triglyceride in the blood), obesity and insulin resistance. This syndrome starts from obesity and accumulation of fat in the abdomen. The fats in the abdomen are triglycerides which is usually associated with CHD (coronary heart disease). The accumulation of fats produces tissue resistance to the actions of insulin. The pancreas compensates by increasing the production of insulin. The overproduction of insulin causes a spike in the blood glucose levels. The higher levels of insulin in the blood promote an increase in the production of triglycerides in the liver. Diabetes results when the insulin produce by the pancreas is not coping with insulin resistance in the tissues. Insulin increases the activity of the sympathetic nervous system and causes the retention of sodium in both kidneys. These eventually result in elevated blood pressure. The combination of disorders in this syndrome may precipitate MI (myocardial infarction) and diseases affecting the heart.

Genetics and research had shown that mutations in the gene pool can result in inheriting essential type hypertension. Further research is being undertaken to determine how these genes play a role in the development of hypertension. Aging is also considered as a cause of hypertension. Though it is a natural occurrence to all of us, the aging process makes the blood vessels loose their ability to be flexible resulting to an elevated blood pressure. A sedentary lifestyle causes hypertension due to lack of physical activity and regular exercise. It is also a lifestyle that can lead to other diseases such as cardiovascular diseases and depression.

Obesity is another cause of hypertension. It is a medical condition wherein the accumulation of fats may have an adverse effect on a person's health. It is defined according to a person's BMI (body mass index). The BMI is obtained by measuring the person's weight in pounds, multiplying it by 703 and dividing it by the product of multiplying height in inches by itself (BMI = weight in lbs X 703 / height in inches x height in inches). A BMI of 25 – 29.9 means the person is overweight, 30- 34.9 means a class 1 obesity, 35 – 39.9 means a class 2 obesity and a BMI greater than 40 means a class 3 obesity. The obvious sign of obesity is the accumulation of fats in the abdomen. Cholesterol and triglyceride levels are typically high and accumulate in the blood vessels. The presence of fats in the blood vessels results to atherosclerosis. Excessive weight gain also increases the pressure on the heart. All of the above and other consequences from obesity elevate the blood pressure.

Bodily diseases as discussed in secondary type hypertension, can itself be a cause of elevated blood pressure. Treating the underlying disease will result in a lower blood pressure. Excessive alcohol intake can be attributed to a drinking habit or alcoholism. Alcohol in large quantities elevates the blood pressure and chronic use will damage the various tissues of the body including the nervous system.

Smoking tobacco and cigarettes are a recreation found enjoyable by some people. Chronic smokers are addicted to the nicotine substance in tobacco or cigarette. Nicotine is absorbed quickly in the lungs through the blood vessels and travels to the brain. It produces euphoria and relaxation. Smoking causes vascular stenosis (narrowing of the blood vessels) or hardening of the blood vessels and other diseases such as lung cancer, myocardial infarction, stroke and impotence. Blood pressure is elevated because of the stimulation of the nervous system and constriction of the blood vessels.

Stress is another cause of hypertension. The occurrence of stress is universal. It is a feeling of strain and pressure from events of daily life. It can be positive, sometimes termed "eustress" if it is moderate, depending on the degree of and the individual's perception of stress. A negative impact results in anxiety, depression, exhaustion, headaches, gastrointestinal disturbances, and among others. A stressful lifestyle producing adrenalin rush and intense encounters elevates blood pressure.

The body's response to stress comes in 3 stages: alarm, resistance and exhaustion. The initial response of the body to stress is the alarm stage. It consists of hyperarousal of the sympathetic nervous system that releases hormones such as cortisol and adrenaline. There is a boost in energy, muscles are tensed, the heart beats faster, veins are constricted and blood pressure is elevated. Emotionally and cognitively a "fight or flight" response occurs. In the resistance stage, the body makes attempts to resist the stressor. Then the energy levels and the intensity of the body's reaction begin declining. Finally the body gets to the exhaustion stage in attempts to resist the stress. The desire and motivation for doing normal daily activities of living become minimal. Energy is drained leading to tiredness and fatigue. Exhaustion continues until the stressor is finally removed and resolved. The effect of stress on the body if unresolved can be fatal. It often results in heart diseases and mental disorders as well as high blood pressure among other negative effects.

Certain types of drugs and medications as discussed under secondary hypertension produce an elevated blood pressure. PPA (phenylpropanolamine) medication and the class of decongestants such as pseudoephedrine, tetrahydrolizine and phenylephrine elevates blood pressure. These drugs enhance the actions of both epinephrine and norepinephrine resulting to vasoconstriction. Antidepressants such as MAO (monoamine oxidase) and TCA (tricyclic antidepressant) have direct effects on the nervous system causing an increase in heart rate and an elevated blood pressure. Ephedra supplement for weight loss has sympathomimetic qualities that stimulate catecholamines resulting in hypertension. Amphetamines stimulate the nervous system causing vasoconstriction, tachycardia, palpitation and among other adverse effects. Herbal supplements such as yohimbe, though often believed safe by the layperson due to their "natural" labeling, also stimulate the release of catecholamines that increases adrenergic activity also potentially resulting in tachycardia, hypertension and agitation.

Dietary intake of excess sodium promotes an increase in the intravascular fluid volume. Through the process of osmosis, fluid is attracted and retained by the sodium element increasing the volume of fluid. The increase in the intravascular fluid volume leads to an increase in the cardiac output and peripheral resistance resulting in an elevated blood pressure. Constant intake of excessive salt over time results not only in hypertension but also in strokes and cardiovascular diseases.

Hypertensive Crisis

Hypertensive crisis is the late stage of hypertension wherein symptoms are evident and severe causing damage to one or more organs in the body. The systolic pressure is greater than or equal to 180 mmhg and the diastolic pressure is greater than or equal to 120 mmhg. There are two known types of hypertensive crisis; malignant hypertension and hypertensive urgency. Malignant hypertension is also known as hypertensive emergency. The symptoms are severe and intolerable headache, bilateral papilledema (swelling of optic discs of both eyes), retinal hemorrhage (bleeding in the retina), vomiting, hematuria (blood in the urine), dyspnea (shortness of breath), epistaxis (nose bleeding), severe symptoms of anxiety, chest pain and seizures among others. Hypertensive urgency does not have severe symptoms that indicate organ damage but can become malignant if not attended or treated within 24 – 48 hours. The typical symptoms are headache and epistaxis.

The immediate treatment for a malignant hypertension is an intravenous sodium nitroprusside injection. This medication will lower the blood pressure through its nitric oxide compound by relaxing the smooth muscles of the blood vessels and reducing peripheral resistance. It reduces the preload and afterload of the heart. If this drug is not available, clonidine and captopril can be use. The goal of treating malignant hypertension is to lower the blood pressure not more than 25 % for the first hour and gradually decreasing it thereafter. This is to allow the body organs to adjust and avoid a sudden impact of lowered blood pressure which could compromise blood flow.

The complications of hypertensive crisis are cerebrovascular accident (stroke), oss of consciousness, amnesia (memory loss), myocardial infarction (heart attack), renal failure, pulmonary edema, numbness, weakness, lumbar pain (back pain), angina (chest pain), among others.

Complications of Uncontrolled Hypertension

The complications from hypertension are developed over time. It may lead to a hypertensive emergency. Prolonged hypertension results to the injury of the wall of the blood vessel. It damages the various organs of the body such as the eyes, kidneys, heart, brain and the arteries.

The eyes have tiny blood vessels that are easily injured. Hypertension causes injury by vasoconstriction, sclerosis and blockage in the flow of blood. Too much pressure in the retinal arteries causes scarring and hemorrhages. Exudates eventually leak from retinal arteries and swelling of the optic disc persists. This pathological damage to the retina is called hypertensive retinopathy.

The kidneys have small arteries that carry oxygenated blood. Hypertension damages these blood vessels. In effect it disrupts the blood flow to the entire kidney. The function of the kidney will be impaired resulting to accumulation of waste products in the body.

Severe kidney damage results to renal failure. Dialysis and kidney transplant are possible treatments.

The heart pumps the oxygenated blood to the arteries for distribution throughout the body. The heart also receives blood from the coronary artery. Hypertension causes atherosclerosis of the coronary artery that can limit the oxygenated blood supply to the heart. When this happens, angina pectoris (chest pain) is a resultant symptom. Furthermore, the arteries in the different parts of the body are narrowed causing the heart to pump harder. When the heart pumps harder it thickens and increases the size of the left ventricle. This is called left ventricular hypertrophy. The hypertrophy can lead to heart failure and heart attacks.

The brain has arteries that supply blood to its different parts. Hypertension causes the narrowing of the cerebral arteries. Atherosclerotic plaques develop overtime and a blood clot may form. This results in a blockage in the blood flow and an immediate ischemic stroke. The blood vessel can also rupture causing a hemorrhagic stroke. The brain tissue is damaged, often severely, in both conditions.

The walls of the arteries are considered elastic but hypertension accelerates the progression of atherosclerosis. In atherosclerosis; the cholesterol, fibrous tissues and calcium form a plaque attached to the wall constricting the diameter of the vessel and limiting the blood flow to the different organs of the body. There are also areas of the blood vessel that are weakened and an excess pressure will create a bulge called an aneurysm. The rupture of an aneurysm can occur at anytime; it is most likely to be fatal if it was formed in the aorta.

To prevent the complications of hypertension; screening, monitoring and appropriate management is necessary. Compliance to a prescribed regimen is needed for an effective treatment process. Refer to the discussion in Chapter 8 of this book.

Chapter 6 Low Blood Pressure: Facts About Hypotension

The state of hypotension is a lowered blood pressure in the arteries. It is a physiological event rather than a psychological one. The blood pressure reading is usually less than 90 mmhg for the systolic pressure and less than 60 mmhg for the diastolic pressure.

Causes of Low Blood Pressure

Hypotension is caused by certain factors and conditions such as pathological heart conditions, disorders in the endocrinary glands, a low blood volume, antihypertensive medications, vasodilation and immobilization.

Certain pathological heart conditions like a defective heart structure causes hypotension. The defective heart structure impedes the ability of the heart to pump blood resulting to a low blood pressure. An incompetent heart valve for instance will cause a backflow of blood and insufficient cardiac output will be the aftermath. As a consequence, an inadequate amount of blood is distributed to the various organs rendering their function insufficient resulting to a number of symptoms. The other heart conditions that cause hypotension are severe congestive heart failure, large myocardial infarction and extreme tachycardia.

Disorders and diseases in the endocrinary glands lower the blood pressure through the effects of the hormones. Some of these endocrinary disorders are hypopituitarism (insufficient secretion of the pituitary gland), hypothyroidism (insufficient secretion of the thyroid gland), Addison's disease, hypoglycemia (low blood glucose) and hypoparathyroidism (insufficient secretion of the parathyroid gland).

A low blood volume is another cause for the blood pressure to drop. A sufficient volume of blood is needed to maintain the perfusion of the different organs of the body. The common causes of low blood volume are hemorrhage, starvation, severe diarrhea and vomiting. Inadequate vascular volume will not provide a sufficient supply of oxygenated blood to the various organs resulting to an array of symptoms. Some of these symptoms are weakness, easy fatigability, lack of energy, blackouts, and dizziness among others.

The intake of antihypertensive medications also of course lowers blood pressure. These types of medications slow the heart rate and decrease the pumping ability of the heart. Overdosing from antihypertensive medications can result in loss of consciousness and be fatal.

The excessive dilation of the blood vessels causes hypotension. It does not promote an effective flow of blood. The effect is less perfusion of the different organs of the body. Some of the common causes of excessive vasodilation are sepsis (bacterial infection), acidosis, nitrate medications and anesthetic agents. Brain injury also causes excessive vasodilation because the input of the sympathetic nervous system is reduced resulting to an increase in stimulation by the parasympathetic nervous system of the blood vessels.

Immobilization is another cause for hypotension. Immobilization is the inability to get out of bed because of certain body conditions. These will result in insufficient blood circulation throughout the body. With less oxygenated blood, the body's organs are compromised.

Symptoms of Hypotension

The symptoms of hypotension are dizziness, lightheadedness, syncope (fainting), inability to concentrate, blurring of vision, nausea, cold skin and tachypnea (rapid shallow breathing). These symptoms are the aftermath of insufficient blood flow to the various organs in the body. The cardinal signs are dizziness and lightheadedness.

Orthostatic hypotension or postural hypotension is a drop in the blood pressure when a person suddenly changes position from sitting to standing. In this condition, it is believed that the pool of blood in the extremities during a reclined or sitting position is compromised causing a lesser venous return to the heart. This results in decreased cardiac output and lowered arterial resistance. A test is done to get an accurate blood pressure reading when a person sits, reclines and stands. A drop in 20 mmhg of the systolic pressure and 10 mmhg in the diastolic pressure will confirm a diagnosis of orthostatic hypotension.

Orthostatic hypotension is caused by antihypertensive medications, antidepressants, antipsychotic and antiparkinson drugs. It is also caused by dehydration, fatigue, starvation, diseases of the nervous system and alcoholism. Orthostatic hypotension usually causes accidental falls. The older adult population has a greater number of cases of fall incidents related to orthostatic hypotension than the younger population.

There are times when the body is injured or compromised. Compensatory mechanisms are automatic. The body's attempt to maintain homeostasis sometimes causes a sudden drop in the blood pressure. This condition is usually cause by hemorrhage, septic shock, anaphylactic shock, hypothermia and severe dehydration. Quick intervention is a must to correct the situation.

Chapter 7 Measuring Your Own Blood Pressure

Monitoring and measuring blood pressure at home may not be an easy task for some people even though the procedure itself is not complicated. There will be false readings because of errors but constant practice makes it more accurate. Stress and denial could also be an impediment to regular monitoring. Doing these measurements at home enables a person to participate in his or her own care. A common practice is to consistently do it 15 - 30 minutes after waking up. Measuring blood pressure throughout the day and unto the evening is also a good practice to detect any fluctuation.

Monitoring Blood Pressure Using Either A Mercury Or An Aneroid Blood Pressure Monitor

There are at least three common instruments that can be used in measuring blood pressure at home. These are the mercury blood pressure monitor, aneroid blood pressure monitor and the electronic blood pressure monitor. The first two devices frequently require a second person to perform the procedure. The electronic device is the easiest to use and does not require a second person. Any type of BP monitoring device should be calibrated, functional and within the standards prescribed by the physician.

There has been a controversy using the mercury based blood pressure monitor because of the toxicity of the mercury content in the sphygmomanometer. A concern is that it may leak or spill at some point and causing mercurial pollution in the environment. Another concern is the possibility that mercury will produce damages to the brain and kidneys if it is inhaled or touched. The reaction to this concern is the development of aneroid and electronic blood pressure monitors.

The Procedure for Taking Blood Pressure using a Mercury and Aneroid Blood Pressure Monitor

The equipment needed for this procedure is the stethoscope and mercurial or aneroid blood pressure monitor. Make sure that both are not malfunctioning. The person to be monitored should refrain from any activity such as eating, drinking, exercising, bathing and smoking for at least 30 minutes before the procedure. Such activities will elevate the blood pressure. Avoid taking BP measurements during stress because it raises blood pressure. All tight fitting clothes should be removed to avoid constriction. If possible sit in a chair with the feet flat on the floor. The arm should be rested in such a way that the cuff is at the level of the heart. Do not talk or make any movement while the measurement of blood pressure is being done.

Consider which arm is best and avoid injured or swollen areas. Select an appropriate cuff size for the arm to prevent erroneous results. Move any clothing away from the arm to ensure accurate measurement. Position the arm at the level of the heart and extend the elbow. Make sure that the palm is turned upward.

Check again to make sure that the BP monitor is not malfunctioning. The pump valves should move freely. Locate the brachial artery by palpating for a pulse in the antecubital space between the arm and the forearm. Once the pulse is located, designate this place for placing the stethoscope. Apply the BP cuff snugly over the upper arm. The placement of the cuff should be at least 1 inch above the antecubital space. The center of the BP cuff should be over the place where the pulse was palpated. The mercury monitor should be placed vertically at eye level.

For an aneroid BP monitor, place the dial gauge at eye level. Turn the valve clockwise to close it then compress the bulb to inflate the cuff to 30 mmhg above the point where the palpated pulse disappears. Deflate the cuff and note the pulse when it is read again. This will provide an estimate of the maximum pressure that is required in measuring the systolic pressure. Insert the earpiece of the stethoscope to both ears and relocate the pulse. Place the diaphragm of the stethoscope directly over the pulse. The entire chest piece should not touch the BP cuff. Turn the valve clockwise to close it then compress to inflate the BP cuff. Inflate until the manometer registers 30 mmhg beyond the point where the pulse was identified or when it was felt when it returned. Slowly deflate the cuff at a rate of 2 – 3 mmhg. This is done to accurately note and hear the Korotkoff's sounds. Take note of the point in the meter gauge where the first sound is heard. This is the diastolic reading. Continue deflating the cuff and take note of the last sound that is heard. This will be the diastolic reading. Deflate the cuff completely to release the trapped vessels and prevent numbness and tingling sensations.

The Procedure for Taking Blood Pressure using an Electronic Blood Pressure Monitor

The same preparatory procedure such as refraining from activities and positioning the arm applies in using the electronic BP monitor. Make sure to understand the parts and functionality of the device. Ensure that it is not malfunctioning. Variations in the operating instructions differ from one device to another. There is a handbook that explains the procedures and the various parts of the electronic BP monitor. Getting familiar with all the information in the handbook is essential for getting accurate results.

The initial step is to check that the parts of the equipment are securely attached to each other such that the air plug is securely inserted in the main unit. Remove tight fitting garments on the upper arm. Sit on a comfortable chair with the feet flat on the floor. This is to enable the body to relax and promote blood circulation. Place the arm on the table with the cuff at the level of the heart. This is done to stabilize the pressure in the arteries and prevent fluctuations in the blood pressure. Hold the grip on the cuff and place the thumb on the thumb grip. Turn the palm upward. Apply the cuff making sure that the blue strip is on the inside of the arm and aligned with the middle finger. The air tube should run down the inside of the arm. Make sure that the bottom of the cuff is approximately 1 inch above the elbow. Wrap the BP cuff firmly around the arm using the cloth strip. Press and hold the start button then release. The cuff will inflate automatically. After a short period inflation will stop and the measurement starts. After completion, the reading appears on the display. It contains the systolic and diastolic pressure as well as the pulse. For most devices the results are stored in the memory of the device and can be accessed at any time following the manufacturer's instruction.

The current normal range in BP measurement is 119 mmhg for the systolic pressure and 80-89 mmhg for the diastolic pressure. There are people who consistently read slightly above or below the range. This type of reading needs to be verified at the physician's office. A reading of 120 – 139 mmhg for the systolic pressure and 80-89 mmhg for the diastolic pressure mean that a person has prehypertension. For most people this is a starting point for lifestyle modification. A reading of 140 – 159 mmhg for the systolic pressure and 90-99 mmhg for the diastolic pressure means that a person has stage 1 of hypertension. An antihypertensive medication such as a diuretic is usually prescribed at this point together with lifestyle modification. A reading of 160 mmhg for the systolic pressure and 100 mmhg for the diastolic pressure means that the person has a stage 2 hypertension. A more intensive medication regimen such as combination drugs is prescribed in this stage. Dosages are usually adjusted to bring the blood pressure to a lower reading. Finally a reading of 180 mmhg for the systolic pressure and 110 mmhg for the diastolic pressure means that a person is in hypertensive crisis. At this point, the physician would require the person to be treated in a hospital to avoid organ damages.

In cases of a reading below 100 mmhg for the systolic pressure, there is often an accompanying symptom that will trigger the person to seek professional help and even call 911 for emergency. If the person is incapacitated, it is usually the other members of the household that would seek emergency help.

Chapter 8 Blood Pressure Management

When a person participates in his or her own health care, managing effective care becomes easier. It also creates a more positive outcome. Initially it is a difficult task because of the medical terminologies and complexities of the healthcare system, but exploration and guidance will eventually bring a better understanding.

After the discovery of either an elevated or lowered blood pressure, a person will be encouraged to participate in self-care. The health teaching from a healthcare provider will guide the person in monitoring their blood pressure, managing dietary intake, adhering to a medication regimen, performing exercises and making helpful lifestyle changes.

Managing Dietary Intake

A dietary intake of low sodium is the best and safest start to preventing further elevation in blood pressure. Certain foods such as ketchup, chips, cold cuts, bacon, cheese and canned goods contain a large quantity of salt. Always read the label for the sodium content of any food that is to be eaten. Stay away from table salt and use salt substitute instead. If intake of salt is unavoidable, maintain the recommended intake of 1.5 g per day at the most. Use spices to add more flavor to the food. A DASH (dietary approaches to stop hypertension) diet has been recommended by some organizations. The DASH diet emphasizes an intake of fruits, vegetables, whole grain and low fat dairy foods. Make sure to eat plenty of potassium rich foods such as bananas to control hypertension. Cut down the intake of saturated fat and total fat as a whole.

Managing A Physically Active Body

A person with hypertension is encouraged to be physically active. Upon recommendation from the physician, certain types of exercises will be suggested. Daily or regular exercises promote blood circulation and optimal functionality of the different parts of the body. An aerobic exercise such as walking is generally best. Exercises for stretching such as yoga; and muscle strengthening are also helpful.

Perform exercise as you can tolerate initially and then gradually increase the intensity. An exercise of at least 30 minutes per day with moderate intensity could be the most that a person can do. A walk of 10 minute in three bouts can be substituted for persons who are not advised to engage in a more intense exercise. Other suggested exercises are jogging, swimming – which is easy on the joints, bicycling, gym or fitness classes, dancing activities, games and sports. For strengthening exercises in the gym, as people age more repetitions are usually easier to tolerate and less likely to cause any muscle strain than high levels of weight. Make sure to have a medical review from a physician before engaging in any type of exercise. Initially, there will be limitations and restriction in doing exercises. Always maintain a routine schedule and note if there are symptoms that occur while performing the exercise.

Managing Smoking Cessation

It is not an easy task to give up smoking. This habit produces physiological and psychologically dependence on nicotine. Nicotine is absorbed quickly in the lungs and passes the brain barrier within 10 – 20 seconds after inhalation. Once it is in the nervous system, it binds to receptors and stimulates dopamine. The stimulation causes dopamine to elicit euphoria and relaxation for the smoker. Such experience is perceived as soothing and eventually becomes a habit and an addiction. Nicotine also stimulates the nervous system to release epinephrine in the blood causing hypertension and tachycardia.

To initiate the process of smoking cessation, first requires a determination to stop it. An understanding about the consequences of this habit should also be provided. This may have been taught by a physician or other healthcare provider. For heavy smokers, an NRT (nicotine replacement therapy) that comprises such temporary smoking substitutes helpful for tapering off as nicotine patches, gums, lozenges, sprays and inhalers can be prescribed. These medications will deliver smaller nicotine doses and eventually reduce dependence on nicotine. The intake of the prescribed chantix also helps to reduce the urge to smoke. Finally, a smoking cessation group and other community support group has been shown to be effective in helping smoking cessation.

Managing Stress and Pressure in Daily Life

Negative stress is mostly present in the daily life of a person. It is psychological in nature and it results in anxiety, depression and bodily diseases. Stress releases the hormones cortisol and adrenaline. It increases heartbeat and constricts blood vessels. If unresolved, it causes further deterioration in the different organs of the body.

Managing stress will not be easy because it is controlled by the mind and the thinking abilities of the brain. If there is a physical stressor, removal is the initial step. Psychotherapy is beneficial for some people in managing stress. Counseling and guidance will enable the stressed person to reflect and engage in stress reduction techniques. Cognitive therapy is used to enable the person to think rationally about stressful situations. Yoga, meditation and breathing exercises are stress reducing activities that can be used throughout the week when opportunities arise. Social activity will provide diversion and relief from certain stressful situations. Nature and pets also seem to provide relaxation and stress reduction. Art and play therapy can divert attention and develop skills that will rechannel the stress. Exercise, dancing and sports are other activities that can reduce stress. A combination of two or more of these interventions and techniques will reduce if not eliminate stress in a person's life.

Managing Blood Pressure through Medications

Compliance with either prescribed antihypertensive or antihypotensive medications is a must. Two or more drugs are often prescribed. The prescribed medications are essential for controlling the irregularity in blood pressure. Dosage and a frequency are determined by the physician. The goal is to promote the action of the prescribed medication and prevent overdosing. Adherence and compliance is of utmost important to treat the impairment in blood pressure regulation.

These prescribed drugs as discussed in Chapter 4 have side effects. Monitoring and taking notes should be done so that it can be discussed with the physician. This will also help the physician and other members of the healthcare team to adjust the dose and provide more intervention as needed. Other medications that are being taken, such as antidepressant, decongestants, steroids and anti-inflammatory drugs and some non-prescription drugs, must be mentioned to the physician to avoid harmful drug interactions.

There are also people with comorbid conditionwho also have either hypotension or hypertension. These people require a more carefully monitored drug intake. There will be instances when the prescribed set of medication will have an inadequate effect. Such inadequate effects should be carefully examined to determine whether non-adherence to prescribed therapy, undiagnosed underlying condition or undisclosed lifestyle behaviors are causing inadequate improvement.

Managing Weight Loss

Losing weight is outright the biggest hurdle. It is never easy even for people without any body problem. Food intake is one of the primary reasons people gain excess. It has been claimed that calories including particularly sugar and fats as well as salt that was taken in excessive quantities over time created a fatty deposition in different areas of the body. Research also claims that genetics and heredity contributes to obesity. Abdominal increase in girth is the distinct sign that a person is becoming overweight.

To manage weight loss, a diet plan should be developed. Dieting may be done using the food pyramid guide by the US Department of Agriculture or the plate method. Most people don't consider it dieting but rather a healthy food guide. The idea with food pyramid guide or the plate method is to consume sufficient nutritious food with daily recommended allowances for quantities. The principle with most diet plans is either to employ a low consumption of carbohydrates or a low consumption in fats and proteins. There are other diet plans that can be considered such as Atkins, Ornish, Zone, Weight Watchers, Gluten free, Protein Power, Paleo and among others. Assistance may also be found in such commercial or non-profit groups as Overeaters Anonymous or Weight Watchers.

After a diet plan, a regular exercise regimen needs to be implemented. As discussed earlier, always consult with the physician regarding the appropriate exercises that can be performed. Aerobic exercise such as walking is usually recommended. Keep notes about changes in weight and the effect of the weight loss program on the body. Compute the BMI and keep track of changes. Discuss the changes and concerns with the physician.

Managing Alcohol Consumption

There are people who drink alcohol occasionally and would be able to stop it as they wish. There are also people who are addicted to alcohol. Even in small quantities, alcohol elevates the blood pressure. Alcoholism is a bigger picture because of the systemic effect on various organs of the body. There is psychological dependence in the context of alcoholism, which makes it a very hard habit to break. The effect of alcohol is stimulation of the GABA receptor which promotes depression. With heavy consumption, the GABA receptors are desensitized and reduced which results in tolerance of larger alcohol doses and physical dependence.

To manage alcohol consumption with occasional drinkers, limit the intake to two drinks a day for males and one for females. For people who are addicted to alcohol, a determination to stop the intake must come first. It is easy to do with occasional drinkers but the task of a lifetime for people who are addicted to alcohol. Helpful is to eliminate all accessible sources of alcohol at home or in the place of work. Consult a psychotherapist for guidance and counseling. Ask help from family members and friends. Sign in for a support group such as Alcoholics Anonymous (AA) and continuously connect to a sponsor.

Managing Health Information

In the process of gathering information from the physician and other members of the healthcare team, there will be certain words that will be new and hard to comprehend. Take notes, ask questions and do research about the medical terminologies. Laboratory results can also be confusing and further understanding is essential to prevent misconception about the figures in the laboratory reports. The dosage, frequency and side effects of the prescribed medications also need to be explained so that there won't be any doubt and misunderstanding. Update oneself with trends or researches about irregularities in blood pressure and newer medications in the market.

Managing Lifestyle Modification

The process of lifestyle modification includes changes in physical activity and exercise, dieting, smoking cessation, limiting alcohol consumption and destressing. This modification process should be tailored to the person's abilities and needs. Goals should be set realistically and reward oneself for any accomplishment. Always consult with the physician and other members of the healthcare team regarding development and progression. Be open to changes and further modification. Take notes and create a daily journal.

Glossary

ACE inhibitor = a antihypertensive drug that prevent the angiotensin converting enzyme from converting angiotensin 1 to angiotensin 2. This drug produces dilation of the blood vessels.

Addison's disease = a disorder of the adrenal glands in which they do not produce sufficient steroid hormones in the body. It is also known as hypoadrenalism.

Adrenal gland = a gland that is located on top of the kidney. It functions to release hormones such as aldosterone and cortisol in response to stress.

Adrenaline = a hormone and a neurotransmitter that regulates heart rate and blood vessels. It is also called epinephrine.

Aldosterone = a steroid hormone produced by the adrenal glands. It increases water retention and conservation of sodium.

Alpha Blocker = an antihypertensive drug that block the alpha adrenergic receptor of the nervous system.

Anaphylactic shock = a severe allergic reaction that has a rapid onset.

Angioedema = a condition wherein there is rapid swelling of the dermis and subcutaneous tissues of the skin.

Angiotensin = a hormone in the human body that causes the constriction of blood vessels.

Angiotensinogen = a globulin protein that is produced by the liver.

Antidiuretic hormone = a hormone in the body that regulates the retention of water. It is also called vasopressin.

Anuria = the absence or nonpassage of urine due to kidney failure.

Atherosclerosis = a body condition wherein the arterial walls have an accumulation of fatty substances consisting of fats.

Atrial natriuretic peptide = a kind of protein hormone that is released by the heart's muscle. It functions to reduce sodium and water.

Beta blocker = an antihypertensive drug that blocks the beta receptors of the sympathetic nervous system.

Bronchospasm = a condition wherein there is a sudden narrowing of the muscles in the wall of the bronchioles.

Calcium channel blocker = a kind of antihypertensive drug that blocks the movement of calcium in the calcium channels throughout the body.

Cardiac arrhythmia = a condition wherein there is an abnormal electrical charge in the heart resulting in overly fast or slow heartbeat. It is also known as cardiac dysrhythmia.

Catecholamine = a protein compound that acts as neuromodulator as well as a hormone. Examples of catecholamines are epinephrine and dopamine.

Central alpha agonist = an antihypertensive drug that blocks the central adrenergic receptors.

Cerebral cortex = a part of the brain that is composed of neural sheet that covers the cerebrum and the cerebellum.

Cirrhosis = a condition wherein a liver tissue is replaced by a scar.

Congestive heart failure = a condition where the heart is unable to pump sufficient blood to meet the needs of entire body.

Coronary heart disease (CHD) = a disease where the coronary arteries are narrowed.

Corticosteroid = a steroid hormone that is produced in the adrenal cortex.

Cortisol = a steroid hormone that is released by the adrenal gland in response to stress.

Cushing's syndrome = a group of symptoms caused by Cushing's disease and pituitary adenoma.

Dihydropyridine = an antihypertensive drug that serves as a calcium channel blocker.

Endocrine gland = a gland of the endocrinary system that secretes hormones directly into the blood.

Epinephrine = also called adrenaline. Refer to adrenaline.

Epoetin = a drug that increases the levels of red blood cells. It also causes hypertension.

GABA receptor = a kind of receptor that responds to the neurotransmitter gamma aminobutyric acid

Glomerular filtration rate = the rate of filtered fluid through the kidney

Hemorrhage = a condition of blood loss that can when excessive require blood transfusion.

Hormone = a chemical that is released by a gland that sends messages affecting other other parts of the body.

Hypertensive retinopathy = a condition where there is a damage to the retina due to an excessively elevated blood pressure.

Inotropic agents = an agent that changes the force of muscular contractions.

Insulin resistance = a state in which the cells of the body fails to respond to the normal action of insulin.

Ischemic stroke = a kind of stroke that result in a decrease of blood supply to the brain.

Korotkoff sound = a sound that is heard during the measurement of blood pressure. It is named after Dr. Nikolai Korotkoff.

Left ventricular hypertrophy = an increase in the size of the muscle of the left ventricle of the heart

Limbic system = a group of brain structure comprising the hippocampus, amygdale, limbic cortex and fornix and the septum.

Low density lipoprotein = a type of lipoprotein that causes health problems and cardiovascular disease.

Monoamine oxidase Inhibitorm (MAOI) = a drug that inhibits the action of monoamine oxidase. It is used for treating depression but can have problematical interactions with several common foods.

Norepinephrine = a catecholamine that functions as a hormone and a neurotransmitter.

Optic disc = a location in the eye where the optic nerve originates. It is also called the blind spot because there are no rod cones that will respond to light.

Phenylpropanolamine (PPA) = an over the counter drug used as a decongestant for cough and cold. It imitates the effect of epinephrine.

Renal failure = a condition wherein the kidneys fail to remove toxic waste from the body. It is also known as kidney failure.

Renin = an enzyme that cleaves angiotensinogen. It is also known as angiotensinogase.

Parasympathetic nervous system = a division of the autonomic nervous system that functions in opposition to the sympathetic nervous system.

Septic shock = a condition wherein there is severe bacterial infection in the body.

Sympathetic nervous system = a division of the autonomic nervous system that functions for fight and flight response during stressful situation. It also regulates homeostasis.

Tricyclic antidepressant (TCA) = a drug that is used to treat clinical depression. It is named after its three structured atoms.

White coat hypertension = it is a phenomenon wherein a person who undergoes a clinic visit has an elevated blood pressure. It is believed to be caused by anxiety and stress.

References

I would like to express my gratitude to:

Dr Lee Robbins for his support in writing this book.

Anatomy and Physiology, Wiley and Sons, New Jersey, 2007
Atkin's diet resources (books, internet, etc.)
Fundamentals of Nursing 3rd Edition, Mosby, Missouri, 1989
Gerontological Nursing 2nd Edition, ANCC, Maryland, 2009
Medical – Surgical Nursing 8th Edition, Lippincott, Pennsylvania, 1996
NCLEX PN, Saunders, Missouri, 2003
NCLEX RN, Mosby, Missouri, 1999
Pathophysiology of Disease 2nd Edition, Appleton and Lange, 1997
Pharmacology in Nursing 21st Edition, Mosby, Missouri 2001
The Johns Hopkins Consumer Guide to Medical Tests, Medletter Associates Inc, New York, 2001
The Johns Hopkins White Papers, Hypertension and Stroke, Medletter Associates Inc, New York, 2003
Wikipidea Free Internet Dictionary

Index

ABPM (ambulatory blood pressure monitoring), 21
ACE inhibitors, 17
adrenal medulla, 13
adrenaline, 23, 32, 37
adverse effects, 5, 16, 17, 18, 19, 23
aerobic exercise, 31
Alcoholics Anonymous (AA), 34
alcoholism, 22, 27, 34
aldosterone levels, 17
Aliskiren, 18
alpha blockers, 17
amiloride, 16
amlodipine, 17
amnesia, 24
Amphetamines, 23
aneroid blood pressure monitor, 28
aneurysm, 25
angina, 24, 25
angioedema, 17
angiotensin 1, 13, 17, 18, 36
angiotensin 2, 13, 17, 18, 36
angiotensin receptor blockers, 18
angiotensinogen peptide, 13
antecubital space, 29
antidiuretic hormones, 13
antihypertensive, 5, 16, 18, 26, 27, 30, 33, 36, 37
anxiety, 17, 21, 23, 24, 32, 39
aorta, 10, 11, 12, 20, 25
arrhythmia, 16, 17, 37
arteries, 10, 11, 15, 20, 24, 25, 26, 29, 37
arterioles, 10, 12, 13
artery, 10, 14, 18, 25, 29
asymptomatic, 5, 18, 19
atenolol, 17
atherosclerosis, 22, 25
Atherosclerosis, 14, 36
atrial natriuretic peptide hormone, 13
atrioventricular valves, 10
autonomic nervous system, 12, 39
autoregulation, 13

azetazolamide, 16
baroreceptors, 12
benazipril, 17
bendroflumethiazide, 16
beta blockers, 17
bicuspid, 10
bilateral papilledema, 24
blood flow, 9, 13, 14, 24, 25, 27
blood pressure, 5, 6, 9, 10, 11, 12, 13, 14, 15, 16, 17, 18, 20, 21, 22, 23, 24, 26, 27, 28, 29, 30, 31, 33, 34, 38, 39
blood pressure monitors, 6, 21, 28
blood pressure regulation, 5, 9, 12, 33
blood vessels, 5, 9, 10, 12, 13, 14, 17, 18, 22, 24, 26, 32, 36
blood volume, 5, 13, 14, 26
BMI (body mass index)., 22
bradycardia, 17
bradykinin, 17
breathing exercises, 32
bronchospasm, 17
calcium channel blockers, 15, 17
capillaries, 5, 10
captopril, 17, 24
carbonic anhydrase inhibitors diuretics, 16
cardiac output, 5, 10, 12, 13, 14, 15, 23, 26, 27
cardiovascular system, 9, 16
carvedilol, 17
catecholamines, 18, 23, 37
Causes of high blood pressure, 21
Causes of low blood pressure, 26
central alpha agonists, 18
cerebrovascular accident, 18, 24
chambers, 9, 10
chantix, 32
CHD (coronary heart disease)., 21
chemoreceptors, 12
cholesterol, 14, 25
Classification of Hypertension, 20
clonidine, 18, 24

41

Cognitive therapy, 32
Complications of Uncontrolled Hypertension, 24
cortisol, 23, 32, 36
DASH (dietary approaches to stop hypertension) diet, 31
deoxygenated blood, 9, 10
diabetes, 4
Diagnosing Hypertension, 21
diastolic pressure, 11, 24, 26, 27, 30
digoxin, 15
dihydropyridines, 17
diltiazem, 17
distal convoluted tubules, 16
diuretics, 16
dizziness, 17, 18, 26, 27
dobutamine, 18
dopamine, 18, 32, 37
dorzolamide, 16
doxazosin, 17
Dry cough, 17
dry mouth, 17, 18
dyspnea, 24
edema, 17, 18
electronic blood pressure monitor, 28
enalapril, 17
Ephedra, 23
ephedrine hydrochloride, 18
epinephrine, 13, 17, 18, 23, 32, 36, 37, 38
epistaxis, 24
Exudates, 24
GABA receptors, 34
gastrointestinal, 16, 17, 18
gastrointestinal disturbances, 23
glomerular filtration rate, 16
headache, 17, 18, 24
healthcare provider, 16, 17, 31, 32
heart, 5, 9, 10, 11, 12, 13, 15, 17, 18, 22, 23, 24, 25, 26, 27, 28, 29, 36, 37, 38
heart attack, 18
hematocrit, 14
hematuria, 24
hemorrhagic stroke, 25
hydralazine, 17
hydrochlorothiazide, 16
hypercalcemia, 16
hyperkalemia, 16, 17, 18
hypertension, 5, 6, 9, 11, 17, 18, 20, 21, 22, 23, 24, 25, 30, 31, 32, 33, 37, 39
Hypertension, 1, 16, 20, 24, 25
Hypertensive crisis, 24
hypertensive emergency, 24
hypertensive retinopathy, 24
hypertriglyceridemia, 21
hyperuricemia, 16
hypokalemia, 16
hyponatremia, 16
hypotension, 6, 9, 11, 16, 17, 18, 26, 27, 33
Hypotension, 1, 26
hypothalamus, 12, 13
hypovolemic shock, 15
insomnia, 17
insulin resistance, 21
kidneys, 13, 16, 22, 24, 28, 38
left atrium, 10
left ventricle, 10, 25, 38
lightheadedness, 27
lisinopril, 17
losartan, 18
low cardiac output, 15
low density lipoproteins, 14
lumbar pain, 24
lungs, 10, 22, 32
Malignant hypertension, 24
Managing A Physically Active Body, 31
Managing Alcohol Consumption, 34
Managing Blood Pressure through Medications, 33
Managing Dietary Intake, 31
Managing Health Information, 34
Managing Lifestyle Modification, 35
Managing Smoking Cessation, 32
Managing Stress and Pressure in Daily Life, 32
Managing Weight Loss, 33
MAO (monoamine oxidase), 23
medulla oblongata, 12
mercury blood pressure monitor, 28
mercury sphygmomanometer, 21
metabolic acidosis, 16

Metabolic Syndrome, 21
methyldopa, 18
metoprolol, 17
minoxidil, 17
mmhg, 20, 21, 24, 26, 27, 29, 30
muscle cramps, 16
myocardial infarction, 18, 22, 24, 26
myocardial ischemia, 18
negative inotropic agents, 15
neural receptors, 5, 12
neurotransmitter, 14, 36, 37, 38
nicardipine, 17
Nicotine, 22, 32
noradrenaline hydrotartrate, 18
norepinephrine, 13, 14, 18, 23
NRT (nicotine replacement therapy), 32
orthostatic hypotension, 6, 16, 27
oxygenated blood, 10, 24, 25, 26, 27
oxygenation, 10
palpitation, 18, 23
panic disorders, 17
parasympathetic, 12, 27
peripheral resistance, 5, 14, 17, 18, 20, 23, 24
phenylephrine, 18, 23
plate method, 33
positive inotropic, 15
postural hypotension, 16, 27
potassium sparing diuretics, 16
Primary hypertension, 20
proprioceptors, 12
proximal tubules, 16
Psychotherapy, 32
Pulmonary circulation, 10
pulmonary edema, 24
pulmonary vein, 10
pulmonic, 10
renal failure, 24, 25
renin, 13
renin inhibitor, 18
renin-angiotensin-aldosterone hormonal system (RAAS), 13
retinal hemorrhage, 24
right atrium, 9, 10
right ventricle, 10
Secondary hypertension, 20
semilunar valves, 10
silent killer, 20
Smoking, 22
sodium, 13, 16, 22, 23, 31, 36
sodium nitroprusside, 24
sphygmomanometer, 28
spironolactone, 16
sternum, 9
stress, 5, 6, 17, 21, 22, 23, 28, 32, 36, 37, 39
stressful lifestyle, 23
stroke, 18, 22, 24, 25, 38
sympathetic, 12, 13, 14, 17, 18, 22, 23, 27, 36, 39
sympathomimetics, 18
Symptoms of Hypotension, 27
systemic circulation, 10
systolic pressure, 11, 24, 26, 27, 29, 30
tachycardia, 17, 18, 23, 26, 32
tachypnea, 27
TCA (tricyclic antidepressant), 20, 23
terazosin, 17
tetrahydrolizine, 23
The Procedure for Taking Blood Pressure using a Mercury and Aneroid Blood Pressure Monitor, 28
The Procedure for Taking Blood Pressure using an Electronic Blood Pressure Monitor, 29
theobromine, 16
theophylline, 16
thoracic cavity, 9
triamterene, 16
tricuspid, 10
triglycerides, 14, 21
valsartan, 18
valves, 9, 10, 15, 29
vascular stenosis, 22
vascular volume, 26
vasoconstriction, 13, 20, 23, 24
vasodilation, 13, 17, 18, 26
vasodilators, 17
vasopressin, 13, 36
vasopressors, 18
veins, 9, 10, 11, 23
ventricles, 9, 10, 14

venules, 10
verapamil, 17
viscous, 14
volume of blood, 13, 14, 15, 26

vomiting, 16, 17, 24, 26
White coat hypertension, 21
xanthine diuretics, 16

***Kindly write a review about this book to help other readers that could benefit from this text. Thank you.

And please feel free to browse my other books @ Amazon.com

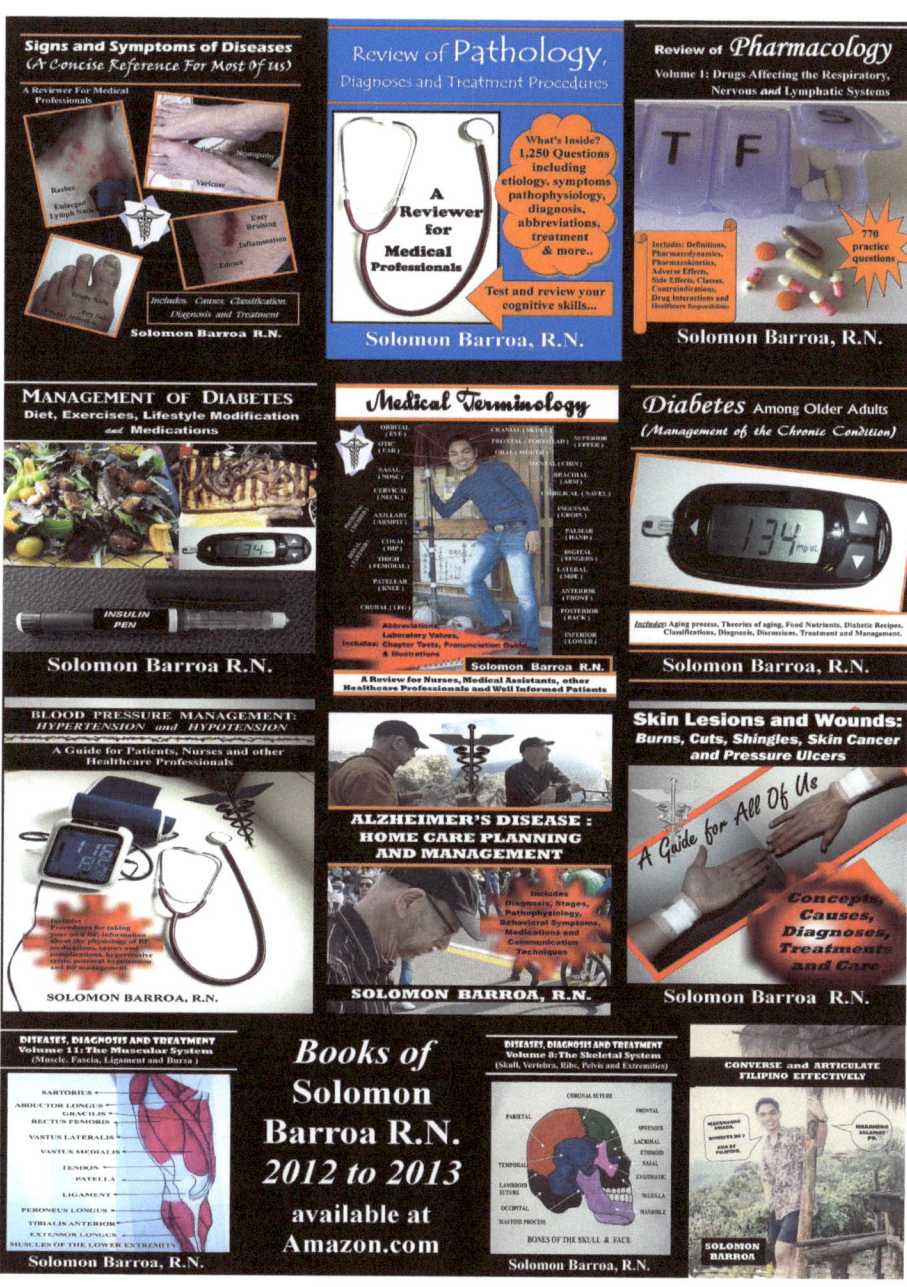

Connect with me online :

Facebook: http://www.facebook.com/solomon.barroa
Twitter: https://twitter.com/solomonbarroa
Amazon: amazon.com/author/solomonbarroa
LinkedIn: http://www.linkedin.com/in/solomonbarroa

 www.ingramcontent.com/pod-product-compliance
Lightning Source LLC
Chambersburg PA
CBHW050830180526
45159CB00004B/1849